RRT® Board Exam Series

Dominate the Airway Management Portion of the Respiratory Therapy Board Exam

By Damon Wiseley B.H.S.c., RRT

www.respiratorytherapyprograms.com

RRT® Board Exam Series

Dominate the Airway Management Portion of the Respiratory Therapy Board Exam.

Copyright © Wiseley LLC 2016

Table of Contents

Part 5: Airway Clearance Techniques

Bronchial Hygiene Devices & Maneuvers
Postural Drainage
Manual Percussion/Chest Physiotherapy
Vibratory PEP
HFCWO
Insufflation/exsufflation device
Huff cough maneuver
Quad cough maneuver
Mucolytics
Suctioning
Heat & Humidification
Bronchoscopy
Mucous Shaver

Part 6: Airway Emergencies Common to Children
Foreign Body Airway Obstruction
Epiglottitis
Croup

Part 7: RRT Exam Practice

Exam Tips Summary

Practice Questions

Practice Questions With Rationales

About the Exam

The National Board for Respiratory Care (NBRC) awards the Registered Respiratory Therapist (RRT) credential to graduates of accredited respiratory therapy programs that meet the following criteria:
1. Pass the Therapist Multiple Choice (TMC) exam high cut mark
2. Pass the Clinical Simulation Exams (CSE)
3. Meet all other NBRC eligibility requirements.

TMC exam candidates are given 3 hours to complete the 160 questions. Twenty questions are under review for future exams and will not count towards your final score. The cost of the TMC is $190. The TMC exam consists of a low cut score and a high cut score. Candidates who achieve a high cut score on the TMC exam are invited to take the Clinical Simulation Exam (CSE).

The CSE exam includes 22 questions. Two of these questions are under review for future exams and will not count towards your final score.

Unfortunately, the high cut score is known only to the National Board for Respiratory Care (NBRC) and remains unpublished. The cost of the CSE exam is $200.

One thing we know is missing the cut will cost you an additional $150 to retake the TMC-RRT exam. Failing the CSE is also costly, as the price remains $200 no matter how often you attempt it.

Important note: If you do not make the high cut on the TMC, but pass the low cut you will earn your CRT. However, you cannot take the CSE exam until you first retake the TMC exam and pass the high cut mark. Then, you must still pass the CSE to be awarded the RRT credential.

About this Book

Congratulations on purchasing this book and committing to making the high cut on the RRT board exams! Taking the RRT board exams can be an intimidating process for those who are not prepared.

This book aims to increase your exam confidence level by preparing you for the airway management portion of the TMC-RRT and CSE exams. I've tried to add as much value as possible, while also being careful to not overwhelm you with too much information.

The _MOST_ important tools this book will give to you are:

> ➤ **A thorough review of airway management**
> ➤ **The ability to connect airway management content to specific questions you may encounter on the TMC-RRT and clinical simulation exams.**
> ➤ **Recommendations based on common airway management problems**
> ➤ **Practice exam questions with thorough rationales for each correct and incorrect answer**
> ➤ **Practice questions based on the newest and most current NBRC testing matrix**

Opening The Airway

Loss of muscle tone in the unconscious patient causes the base of the tongue to obstruct the airway. <u>This is the most common cause of airway obstruction.</u> Performing the head-tilt/chin lift or jaw thrust maneuver can reopen the airway.

Head-tilt/chin-lift
The head-tilt/chin-lift method is the preferred method of establishing an airway during CPR.

Exam tip: Do not perform if spinal trauma suspected. For example, motor vehicle accidents, falls

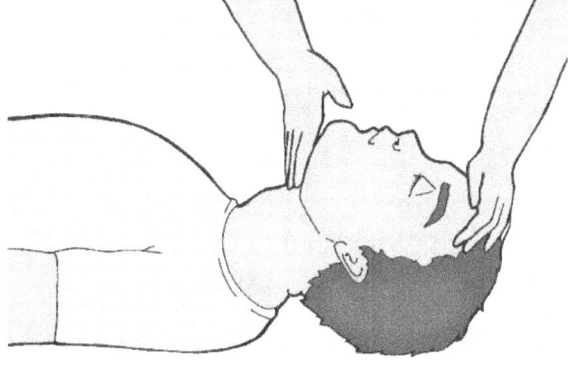

Jaw thrust
The traditional jaw thrust maneuver opens the airway by slightly extending the neck and moving the jaw anteriorly. Neck extension is undesirable in patients with suspected cervical injury. The modified jaw thrust is preferred in such cases.

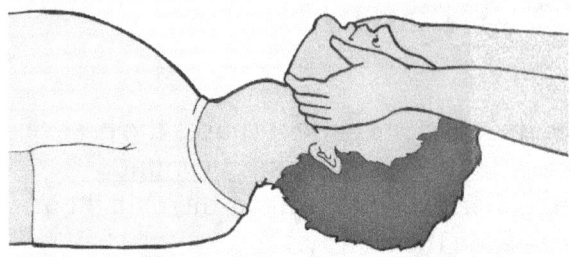

Modified Jaw Thrust

The modified jaw thrust moves the jaw anteriorly without extending the neck. To perform the modified jaw thrust maneuver you must position yourself behind the head of the patient. Place the tips of your fingers under the patient's mandible and move it up and forward. Perform the jaw thrust maneuver if neck or spinal trauma is suspected.

Practice Question 1

An unconscious patient arrives in the emergency department following a motor vehicle accident. What should the respiratory therapist do FIRST to establish this patient's airway?

    A. Head-tilt/chin-lift maneuver
    B. Modified jaw thrust maneuver
    C. Reposition the patient on their side
    D. Jaw thrust maneuver

Answer

    A. Incorrect. The head-tilt/chin-lift maneuver is contraindicated in patients with possible spinal trauma.
    B. Correct. The jaw thrust maneuver is indicated in patients with possible spinal injury.
    C. Incorrect. Moving a patient with a possible spinal injury is contraindicated.
    D. Incorrect. The jaw thrust maneuver slightly extends the patient's neck. This is contraindicated in a patient with possible spinal trauma. Use the modified jaw thrust maneuver instead.

Pharyngeal Airways

Despite opening the airway using the head-tilt/chin-lift or jaw thrust methods, the base of the tongue may still obstruct the airway. Placing a pharyngeal airway may prevent this from happening. There are two types of pharyngeal airways:

1. Oropharyngeal airways
2. Nasopharyngeal airways

Oropharyngeal Airways

Oropharyngeal airways are placed in the <u>unconscious</u> patient's mouth to prevent the base of the tongue from falling back and obstructing the airway. They can be used while manually ventilating a patient with a bag and mask. Oropharyngeal airways can also be placed in the intubated patient's mouth to protect the endotracheal tube from a patient who is biting.

Exam tip: Do not recommend oropharyngeal airways for conscious or semi-conscious patients as they may cause gagging, vomiting, and/or laryngospasm.

There are two types of oropharyngeal airways

1. **Berman airways** have a hard plastic *exterior* channel to facilitate passing of a suction catheter.

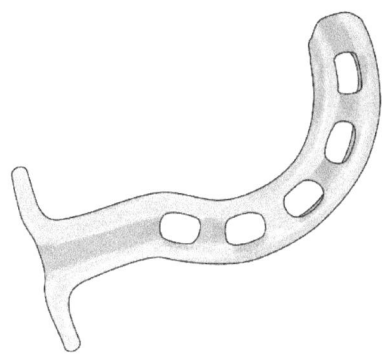

2. **Guedel airways** are soft and pliable. They have an *interior* channel to facilitate passing of a suction catheter.

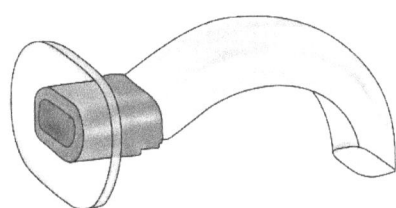

Indications
1. Prevent or treat airway obstruction caused by the base of the tongue in the unconscious, obtunded, or heavily sedated patient.
2. Protect the ETT from biting by orally intubated patients.
3. Facilitate suctioning of the oropharynx.

Complications
1. **Do not use in a conscious patient.**
2. Gagging, vomiting, laryngospasm. <u>Remove the airway immediately</u> if any of these occur.

Insertion Technique
Determine the correct size by measuring from the angle of the jaw to the corner of the mouth. The tip of the airway is first inserted upside down until it reaches the hard palate. Next, it is

rotated 180 degrees as it is advanced over and past the tongue. The tip of the airway should lie at the base of the tongue and above the epiglottis. Care must be taken to not push the tongue further back into the pharynx as this will worsen the obstruction.

Nasopharyngeal Airways

Nasopharyngeal airways can be inserted into the nose of a conscious adult patient. They help reduce trauma to the nasal mucosa of patients requiring frequent nasotracheal suctioning. They also prevent the base of the tongue from falling back and obstructing the airway.

Advantages of Nasopharyngeal Airway
1. Tolerated well by the conscious patient
2. Allows patient to speak, eat, and drink

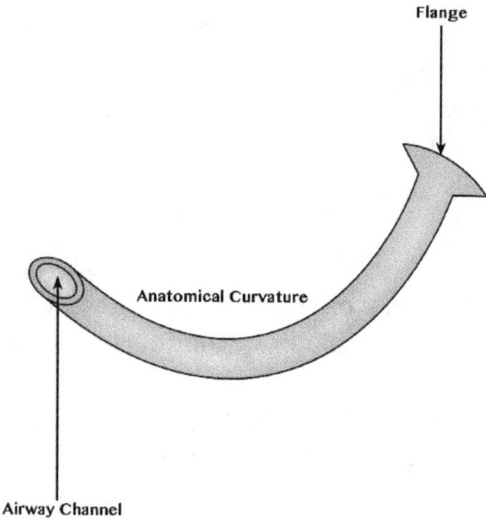

Indications
1. Patients with ineffective cough requiring frequent nasotracheal suctioning.
2. Conscious patient whose tongue is obstructing the airway.

3. Patients requiring a pharyngeal airway, but with conditions that prevent access to the mouth, such as a patient having a seizure.

Complications
1. Epistaxis (nose bleed)
2. Increased airway resistance.
3. Airway obstruction due to plugging of the nasopharyngeal airway with secretions. Change airway every 24 hours.
4. Aspiration of the nasopharyngeal airway. Be sure to use the correct diameter as the airway could be aspirated into the lungs if too small.

Contraindications
1. Closed head injury
2. Patients receiving anticoagulant therapy

Insertion Technique
Determine the correct length by measuring the distance from the patient's earlobe to the tip of their nose. The outer diameter should be equal to the inner diameter of the patient's nares.

1. Use water-soluble lubricant to reduce trauma from insertion.
2. Tilt head slightly backward
3. Slowly advance airway into the right or left nare with airway perpendicular to the patients face and with the bevel facing the septum. The distal tip should rest behind the uvula and the flange should rest outside the nasal opening. **Do not rotate the airway as it is inserted.**
4. Tape may be placed around the flange to secure the airway.

Practice Question 2

An oropharyngeal airway is placed in a lethargic patient to maintain a patent airway. The patient begins to cough and gag. What should the respiratory therapist do NEXT?

    A. Reassure the patient
    B. Continue to monitor the patient
    C. Remove the oropharyngeal airway
    D. Intubate the patient

Answer

    A. Incorrect. Reassuring the patient will have no effect on the patient's gag reflex. Oropharyngeal airways are contraindicated in patients with an intact gag reflex due to the risk of vomiting and aspiration
    B. Incorrect. Monitoring the patient will not address the risk of gagging, vomiting and aspirating caused by the oropharyngeal airway.
    C. Correct. Oropharyngeal airways are contraindicated in patients with an intact gag reflex.
    D. Incorrect. Intubation is not indicated. A nasopharyngeal airway may be placed after removing the oropharyngeal airway.

Practice Question 3

A conscious patient in the ICU has a large amount of secretions requiring frequent nasotracheal suctioning. Which of the following airways should the respiratory therapist recommend?

    A. Berman airway
    B. Tracheostomy tube
    C. Nasopharyngeal airway
    D. Guedel airway

Answer

    A. Incorrect. The Berman oropharyngeal airway is contraindicated in conscious patients.
    B. Incorrect. A tracheostomy tube is not indicated.

C. Correct. A nasopharyngeal airway is well tolerated in a conscious patient and can reduce trauma to the nares from frequent suctioning.
D. Incorrect. The Guedel oropharyngeal airway is contraindicated in conscious patients.

Practice Question 4

Contraindications to nasopharyngeal airway insertion include?

A. Unconscious patient
B. Patient who is eating
C. Closed head injury
D. Excessive bronchial secretions

Answer

A. Incorrect. Nasopharyngeal airways can be tolerated in both conscious and unconscious patients.
B. Incorrect. Patients can still eat with a nasopharyngeal airway in place.
C. Correct. Closed head injuries may be adversely affected by insertion of a nasopharyngeal airway.
D. Incorrect. Patients requiring frequent nasotracheal suctioning would benefit from the placement of a nasopharyngeal airway.

Supraglottic Airways

Supraglottic airways sit just above the glottic opening to the airway. Supraglottic airway devices (SAD) can provide a means of ventilation in the difficult airway patient. They are also popular as a means of short-term ventilation in patients undergoing surgery.

Laryngeal Mask Airway (LMA)

The LMA can provide ventilation in difficult airway cases. Some LMA's allow passage of an endotracheal tube through the LMA itself into the patient's airway.

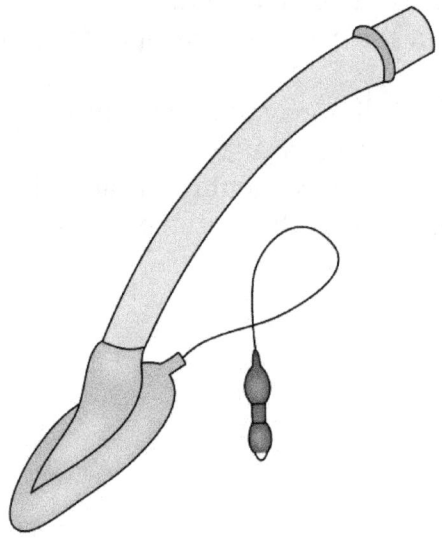

Indications
1. Difficult airway/Failed intubation
2. Difficult to bag/mask ventilate
3. Short-term ventilation when intubation is not necessary during elective surgery.

Contraindications and Disadvantages
1. Do not use if a risk of aspiration exists

2. Do not use if personnel are not trained in LMA insertion
3. <u>The patient must be properly anesthetized to avoid gagging, laryngospasm, and/or vomiting.</u>
4. Ventilation may not be effective if high airway pressures are required, or if the patient has abnormal airway anatomy. High airway pressures may also cause gastric insufflation when using the LMA.

Insertion technique
1. Lubricate the fully deflated cuff
2. Using the index finger, blindly guide the mask into the oropharynx.
3. When in place, inflate the cuff until no leak is heard, or to a maximum of 60 cm H20. Do not overinflate.
4. The LMA can be removed when the patient can open his mouth on command.

King Supraglottic airway

The King airway is a <u>single lumen</u> tube with <u>both a distal and proximal cuff</u>. The distal cuff is **inserted into the esophagus**. The larger, proximal cuff sits above the airway. <u>A single pilot balloon</u> is used to inflate both the distal and proximal cuffs. The cuffs are inflated using the single pilot balloon to either 60 cm H20 or until no leak is heard at peak inspiration.

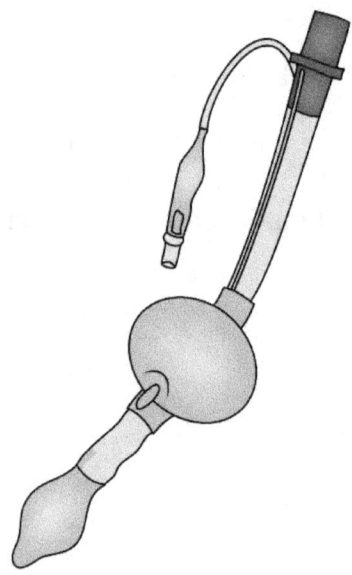

Indications
1. Difficult airway (difficult to bag-mask ventilate, difficult to intubate) in the out of hospital setting.
2. Lack of trained personnel in endotracheal intubation.

Contraindications
1. Conscious patient, intact gag reflex.
2. DNR

Exam Tip: The King airway is not intended for long-term ventilation and should be replaced with an endotracheal tube as soon as possible.

Esophageal Tracheal Combitube (ETC)

The esophageal tracheal combitube (ETC) is so named because it can provide effective ventilation whether placed in the esophagus or the trachea. The ETC has <u>two lumens, two pilot balloons, a large pharyngeal cuff and a smaller esophageal cuff.</u> The ETC is especially useful as a pre-hospital emergency airway.

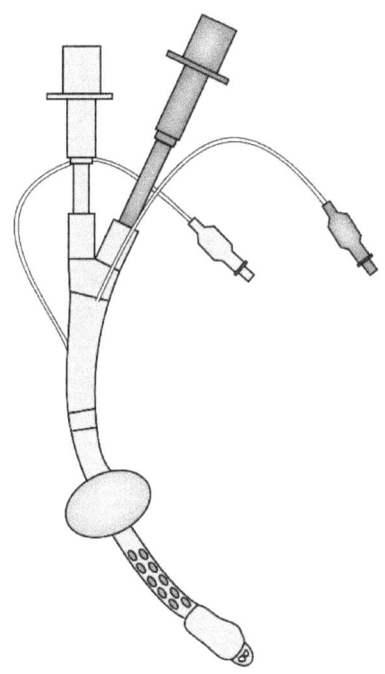

Indications
1. Difficult airway (difficult to bag-mask ventilate, difficult to intubate) in the out-of-hospital setting.
2. Lack of trained personnel in endotracheal intubation.

Contraindications
1. Conscious patient, intact gag reflex
2. DNR/DNI

Key Insertion Steps

1. The ETC is <u>blindly inserted</u> without the use of a laryngoscope.
2. Align the patient's teeth between the two black rings.
3. Inflate the large pharyngeal balloon with 100 cc of air.
4. Inflate the small esophageal balloon with 15 cc of air.
5. Ventilate first through the longer, blue tube and auscultate the stomach and lungs.
6. Switch ventilation to the shorter, white tube if auscultation reveals ventilation of the stomach.

Exam Tip: The ETC is not intended for long-term ventilation and should be replaced as soon as possible in the hospital setting.

Tracheal Tubes

Endotracheal Tubes

Endotracheal tubes include the following features and components.

Cuff

The cuff seals the area around the ETT to allow for positive pressure ventilation and prevent aspiration of secretions.

1. <u>High volume/low pressure cuff</u> – These cuffs cover a larger surface area of the airway while using a lower pressure to create a seal. This type of cuff carries a lower risk of tracheal wall damage as compared to low volume/high pressure cuffs.

2. <u>Low volume/high pressure cuff</u> – These cuffs cover a smaller portion of the airway while using a higher pressure to create a seal. This type of cuff imposes a greater risk of damage to the tracheal wall.

Standard 15 mm hub

This standard sized hub can connect to any bag-device or ventilator circuit.

Radio-opaque line

The radio-opaque line extends across the length of the ETT and is used for imaging identification of ETT placement.

Murphy's eye

The Murphy's eye is a hole near the tip of the endotracheal tube. This additional hole allows ventilation to continue if the opening of the ETT becomes obstructed. For example, if the end of the ETT became lodged against the tracheal wall, ventilation would continue through the Murphy's eye.

Pilot tube and balloon with one-way valve

The pilot tube is used to inflate the endotracheal tube cuff.

Depth and size markings

The size of an endotracheal tube refers to its inner diameter. For example, a size 8.0 ETT refers to the inner diameter of the tube.

CASS Endotracheal Tubes

Continuous Aspiration of Subglottic Secretions (CASS) tubes provide continuous subglottic suction just above the cuff at a recommended pressure of -20 mm Hg. **CASS tubes are used to prevent ventilator-associated pneumonia (VAP).** A popular brand of CASS tube is the High-lo evac tube.

Double-Lumen Endotracheal Tubes

Double-lumen tubes contain two separate lumens, each with its own cuff. This allows independent lung ventilation (ventilation of only one lung or each lung at different volumes or pressures).

Double-lumen tubes may also be referred to as endobronchial tubes or Carlen's tubes.

Indications
1. Surgical procedures such as a lobectomy or pneumonectomy requiring independent lung ventilation.
2. Lung abscess (the double lumen tube protects the good lung from the bad lung).

Practice Question 5
Which of the following airways does not require use of a laryngoscope for insertion?

A. Endotracheal tube
B. Esophageal tracheal combitube
C. CASS tube
D. Double-lumen tube

Answer
A. Incorrect. A laryngoscope is required
B. Correct. The esophageal tracheal combitube is blindly inserted without a laryngoscope.
C. Incorrect. A laryngoscope is required
D. Incorrect. A laryngoscope is required

Practice Question 6

Which of the following airways should the respiratory therapist recommend as part of a hospitals VAP protocol for patients receiving mechanical ventilation greater than 24 hours?

A. Endotracheal tube
B. CASS endotracheal tube
C. Laryngeal mask airway
D. Guedel airway

Answer

A. Incorrect. A standard endotracheal tube is inferior to a CASS tube for the prevention of ventilator-associated pneumonia.
B. Correct. Continuous aspiration of subglottic secretions is a useful tool in the prevention of ventilator-associated pneumonia.
C. Incorrect. Laryngeal mask airways are used for short term ventilation and do not provide continuous aspiration of subglottic secretions.
D. Incorrect. Guedel airways cannot support mechanical ventilation.

Practice Question 7

Which of the following airways have two cuffs?

A. King airway
B. Double lumen airway
C. Esophageal tracheal combitube
D. All of the above

Answer

A. Incorrect. The King airway has two cuffs.
B. Incorrect. The double lumen airway has two cuffs.
C. Incorrect. The esophageal tracheal combitube has two cuffs.
D. Correct. All of these airways have two cuffs.

Tracheostomy Tubes

There are countless varieties and styles of tracheostomy tubes in use today. However, the core purpose and functionality of tracheostomy tubes remains the same. For the purpose of preparing for the boards exams, focus on understanding the basics such as cuffed vs. cuffless, when to use a fenestrated tube and when to remove the tracheostomy tube if an obstruction is suspected.

Indications
1. Patients requiring <u>long term ventilation</u>
2. Emergency airway due to upper airway obstruction
3. Emergency airway for patients with severe maxillofacial trauma
4. Anatomical airway abnormalities
5. Obstructive sleep apnea
6. Protect against aspiration

Advantages
1. Decreased airway resistance and less dead space.
2. Patient can eat (cuff should be inflated when eating)
3. Patient can speak if used with speaking device such as a Passy-Muir valve
4. Patient can be easily reconnected to ventilator as needed

Early Complications (first 24 hours post tracheostomy)
1. Bleeding
2. Pneumothorax
3. Subcutaneous emphysema

Late complications (greater than 2 days post tracheostomy)
1. Tracheomalacia – caused by high cuff pressures.

2. Esophageal tracheal fistula – a hole connecting the trachea to the esophagus.
3. Hemorrhage due to innominate artery fistula
4. Infection
5. Obstruction

Tracheostomy Tube Components

Outer cannula
This is the main part of the tracheostomy tube that remains in the patient's stoma until decannulation. The outer cannula serves as the primary structure of the tracheostomy tube. The cuff and flange are attached to the outer cannula.

Inner cannula

The inner cannula resides inside the outer cannula. The inner cannula, unlike the outer cannula, can easily be removed and cleaned to maintain the patency of the airway. The inner cannula also has a hub that connects to a manual resuscitation bag or a ventilator circuit to provide positive pressure ventilation. Inner cannulas are locked in place to prevent the patient from coughing them out.

Non-disposable inner cannulas should be removed and cleaned as needed with a 50/50 mixture of hydrogen peroxide and water. Prior to re-inserting the inner cannula rinse it with sterile water to remove debris and the hydrogen peroxide.

Obturator
The obturator is used only during initial insertion of the tracheostomy tube. The obturator is placed inside the outer cannula. The obturators rounded tip extends just past the end of the tracheostomy tube to minimize trauma during insertion.

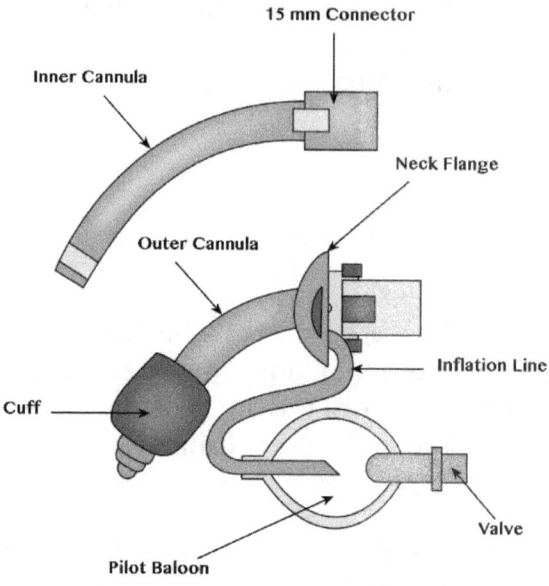

Inner Cannula

15 mm Connector

Neck Flange

Outer Cannula

Inflation Line

Cuff

Pilot Baloon

Valve

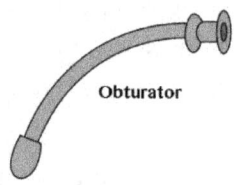

Obturator

Cuff

The tracheostomy cuff can be inflated to seal off the area around the tracheostomy tube when positive pressure ventilation is provided. The cuff should also be inflated when the patient is eating. Maintaining the cuff pressure at safe levels may prevent tracheal wall damage and minimize the risk of silent aspiration.

Three cuff categories

1. High volume/low pressure cuffs (recommended) cause the least damage to the tracheal wall.

2. Low volume/high pressure or tight to shaft cuffs (TTS) are not recommended. These high-pressure cuffs may cause damage to the tracheal wall by exceeding the mucosal capillary perfusion pressure.

3. <u>Foam filled tracheostomy tube cuffs</u> were developed to limit the total pressure applied to the tracheal wall to that of atmospheric pressure. The pilot balloon is left open to air. Foam filled cuffs spontaneously self inflate to seal off air movement around the trachea.

> A major drawback of foam filled cuffs is that they cannot be used with speaking valves because the cuff will not remain deflated. Foam filled cuffs are often referred to by the brand names Bivona and Kamen-Wilkinson.

Exam Tip: A cuff requiring a high amount of pressure to seal the airway may indicate the tracheostomy tube is too small.

Pilot balloon
Air is pushed through the pilot balloon with a syringe to inflate the cuff. The pilot balloon can be connected to a manometer to measure the pressure within the patient's cuff.

Flange
The flange, or neck plate, sits against the patient's neck. Tracheostomy tube ties or sutures are secured to the flange to secure it to the patient. The flange also indicates the inner and outer diameter as well as other special features regarding the tracheostomy tube.

Passy-Muir Speaking valve
The Passy-Muir speaking valve is an optional one-way valve placed on the hub of the tracheostomy tubes inner cannula to allow speech. The patient inhales through the speaking valve, and exhales through their mouth or nose. This allows air to pass through the vocal cords and speech to occur. Passy-Muir valves can be placed on fenestrated or non-fenestrated tracheostomy tubes. **Deflate the cuff before using!**

Special Tracheostomy Tubes

Fenestrated

Fenestrated tracheostomy tubes have a hole near the middle of the tube. The hole, known as a fenestration, allows air to pass through the vocal cords, nose, and mouth when a speaking valve or cap is placed. As a result, the patient can speak and breathe through their nose and mouth. They can also cough secretions into and out of the mouth, the natural way.

Exam Tip: When using a fenestrated tracheostomy tube with a speaking valve or cap, the cuff must be deflated.

Exam Tip: Recommend fenestrated tracheostomy tubes as part of the process of weaning the patient from the tracheostomy tube.

Tracheostomy button

A tracheostomy button is a hollow plastic tube used to keep the stoma open after decannulation. Keeping the stoma open allows a tracheostomy tube to be easily reinserted should the patient not tolerate decannulation. The tracheostomy button can also be used to suction the airway.

The tracheostomy button is cuffless and cannot be used to provide positive pressure ventilation. Tracheostomy buttons are sometimes placed in patients with severe sleep apnea.

Extended length tracheostomy tubes

These extra long tubes are useful for patients with challenging anatomy. They are categorized as either proximal or distal extended length tubes.

1. <u>Proximal</u> extended length tubes are ideal for patients with full or thick necks such as obese patients or those requiring use of a cervical collar.

2. <u>Distal</u> extended length tubes are ideal for patients requiring extra length due to tracheal malacia, stenosis, or granulomas.

Jackson tracheostomy tube

Jackson tracheostomy tubes are made of metal and do not have a cuff. Theses tracheostomy tubes are not encountered very often, however, some long-term tracheostomy patients still use them.

Because they are cuffless, Jackson tracheostomy tubes cannot be used to deliver positive pressure ventilation. The metal composition of these tracheostomy tubes also prohibits their use in MRI. The rigid construction of the Jackson tracheostomy tube does not conform to the patient's anatomy like tracheostomy tubes made of silicone or polyvinyl chloride.

Laryngectomy tubes

A complete or total laryngectomy removes the patient's entire larynx. As a result, a connection from the trachea to the mouth and nose no longer exists.

The patient must permanently breathe through their stoma and can no longer be orally or nasally intubated.

Laryngectomy tubes are shorter than traditional tracheostomy tubes and are always cuffless. Laryngectomy tubes cannot be used to provide positive pressure ventilation.

Practice Question 8
What type of tracheostomy tube should the respiratory therapist select for a patient receiving mechanical ventilation?

    A. Tracheostomy button
    B. Foam filled self-inflating cuff
    C. Jackson tracheostomy tube
    D. Cuffed tracheostomy tube

Answer

A. Incorrect. A tracheostomy button cannot be used to provide positive pressure ventilation.
B. Incorrect. A foam filled self-inflating cuff may not provide an adequate seal to provide positive pressure ventilation.
C. Incorrect. A Jackson tracheostomy tube does not have a cuff. Therefore, positive pressure ventilation cannot be provided.
D. Correct. Mechanical ventilation requires a cuffed tracheostomy tube.

Practice Question 9

A patient with a complete laryngectomy develops severe respiratory distress and requires mechanical ventilation emergently. The patient has a laryngectomy tube in place. What should the respiratory therapist recommend?

A. Intubate the patient orally
B. Intubate the patient nasotracheally
C. Remove the laryngectomy tube and insert a cuffed tracheostomy tube into the stoma
D. Bag-valve mask ventilate the patient until an airway is provided

Answer

A. Incorrect. Patients with a complete laryngectomy lack a connection from the mouth to the trachea.
B. Incorrect. Patients with a complete laryngectomy lack a connection from the nose to the trachea.
C. Correct. A laryngectomy tube maintains the patency of a stoma. As a result, the laryngectomy can be removed and an airway placed into the stoma to provide ventilation.
D. Incorrect. No connection exists from the nose and mouth to the patient's trachea. Therefore, bag-valve mask ventilation will not ventilate the lungs.

Practice Question 10

A late complication of tracheostomy tube placement includes which of the following?

A. Esophageal tracheal fistula
B. Subcutaneous emphysema
C. Tracheomalacia
D. Both A and C

Answer
A. Incorrect. Esophageal tracheal fistula is not the only late complication on this list.
B. Incorrect. Subcutaneous emphysema is not a late complication
C. Incorrect. Trachomalacia is not the only late complication on this list.
D. Correct. Both esophageal tracheal fistula and tracheomalacia are late complications of tracheostomy tube placement.

Manual Resuscitators

The RRT exam will test your knowledge of when and how to correctly use manual resuscitation devices. Several different devices are available to provide manual resuscitation/ventilation.

Bag-Valve Mask (BVM)

Bag-valve mask devices are categorized as either self-inflating or flow-inflating.

Self-inflating devices can deliver positive pressure ventilation with or without connection to a gas source. As a result, these should be **used for patient transport**.

Flow-inflating devices require a continuous flow of gas to deliver a breath. These devices are primarily used in the operating room environment by anesthesiologists. Flow-inflating bags should not be used for transport, as they cannot function if the source gas runs out.

BVM Components (self inflating)

The BVM is made of many key components that must function correctly to be effective.

Bag
The bag itself should self-inflate after being squeezed regardless of whether it is connected to a gas source or not.

Inlet valve
The inlet valve is a one-way valve that allows oxygen into the bag from the reservoir bag or tubing as the bag re-inflates after a breath is delivered.

Exhalation valve
The exhalation valve prevents rebreathing of the patient's exhaled air.

Mask

Must be transparent, capable of creating a seal, have oxygen inlet, and standard 22 mm port for an adult, or15 mm port for infants. Masks come in adult, child, and infant sizes. Some masks are anatomically shaped to fit the contours of the face. Masks are filled with air to create a cushion when applied to the patient's face.

Oxygen reservoir attachment

An oxygen reservoir, in the form of a bag or tubing, should be attached to the self-inflating bag device. The oxygen reservoir fills with pure oxygen between delivery of breaths. When the self-inflating bag re-expands after being squeezed, it draws in a high concentration of oxygen. As a result, a bag with a reservoir can provide a FiO2 level close to 100%. A self-inflating bag device without an oxygen reservoir may only deliver a FiO2 between 40% and 50%.

PEEP valve

Optional spring-loaded valve attaches to the expiratory side of the patient valve.

Pressure relief valve

Pressure relief valves are a safety feature used most often with infant and child bag and mask devices. These valves prevent excessive pressures from being delivered to the patient's lungs.

Pressure manometer

A pressure manometer is a safety feature that may be present on infant bag and mask devices. The pressure manometer gives the therapist a breath-to-breath indication of the peak airway pressures they are applying to the patient.

Exam Tip: Should you troubleshoot a problem with the bag or simply use another manual ventilation device?

Answer: Use another bag or manual ventilation device.

Bag-Valve Mask Ventilation

Bag-valve mask (BVM) ventilation may be more effective when used in conjunction with an oropharyngeal airway. The oropharyngeal airway prevents the base of the tongue from falling back and blocking the airway of the unconscious patient.

Technical key points
1. Set flow 10-15 L/min to achieve highest FiO2 available
2. Insert an oropharyngeal airway in the unconscious patient to prevent the patient's tongue from obstructing the airway.
3. Open the airway using the head-tilt/chin-lift or modified jaw thrust method.
4. Deliver breath over 1 second

Complications
1. Gastric insufflation (Performing the Sellick maneuver may reduce this).
2. Aspiration of gastric contents (Performing the Sellick maneuver may reduce this).
3. Barotrauma

Exam Tip: A BVM is a required piece of equipment when transporting intubated patients and when performing cardioversion.

Exam Tip: If the reservoir bag of the BVM does not refill in between delivered breaths, increase the flow.

Exam Tip: A leak anywhere in the BVM system may cause poor chest rise and/or a lack of resistance when squeezing the bag.

Exam Tip: Remember to use the jaw thrust method if spinal injury is suspected. A patient who fell from a ladder or was involved in a motor vehicle crash may have a spinal injury.

Mouth-To-Valve Mask Device

The mouth-to-valve mask device has a one-way valve and filter to protect the rescuer when delivering breaths. As a result, it reduces the risk of disease transmission and is a safer alternative than mouth-to-mouth.

In addition, supplemental oxygen can be delivered through a port connected to the mask. A FiO2 of up to .50 can be delivered using a mouth-to-valve mask device as compared to only .16 with mouth-to-mouth ventilation.

Pneumatically (Gas) Powered Resuscitators

Advantages
1. Capable of delivering 100% oxygen

Disadvantages
1. Requires a 50 psi gas source to function
2. May cause gastric insufflation.
3. Difficult to assess changes in the patient's lung compliance as compared to a BVM device.
4. May cycle off prematurely when patient is receiving chest compressions.

T-piece Resuscitator

T-piece resuscitators are sometimes favored for use with infants instead of BVM devices due to their consistent application of peak airway pressures and PEEP.

Advantages
Consistent control of peak inspiratory pressure and PEEP
Delivers up to 100% oxygen

Disadvantages
Requires a compressed gas source to operate. Pressures must be set prior to use.

Practice Question 11
The respiratory therapist is transporting an intubated patient to CT-scan using a portable ventilator. The patient is intubated with a size 8.0 ETT secured at 22 cm lip. Which of the following items is most important for the patients transport?

A. Cufflator
B. Bag-valve mask device
C. Additional size 8.0 ETT
D. Laryngeal Mask Airway

Answer
A. Incorrect. A cufflator is not required for transport of the intubated patient.
B. Correct. Due to the high risk of accidental extubation during patient transport, a bag-valve mask is required.
C. Incorrect. An additional airway may be helpful, but is not required during intra-hospital transport.
D. Incorrect. A laryngeal mask airway is not of much use without a bag-valve mask device.

Practice Question 12

Disadvantages of using a pneumatically powered resuscitation device include?

A. Increased likelihood of gastric insufflation
B. Cannot be used for infants
C. Cannot sense changes in the patient's lung compliance
D. All of the above

Answer
A. Incorrect
B. Incorrect
C. Incorrect
D. Correct. These are all disadvantages of using a pneumatically powered resuscitation device.

Management of Acute Airway Obstruction

Be prepared to answer what the therapist should do next, at any point in a choking sequence.

Keys To Exam Success

1. Look for and remove foreign objects from the mouth before ventilating.
2. If alone, perform 2 minutes of CPR before activating the EMS system.
3. Conscious adults get the Heimlich maneuver.
4. Unconscious adults get CPR without checking the pulse.
5. Conscious infants get alternating back blows and chest thrusts (5 each).
6. Unconscious infants get CPR without checking the pulse.

Mild Airway Obstruction

Signs

1. Conscious and responsive
2. Forceful or violent cough
3. Mild stridor

Management

1. Monitor closely and allow them to clear their airway on their own.
2. Activate EMS if the partial obstruction persists or worsens.

Severe Airway Obstruction

Signs

1. Unconscious
2. Cannot cough, talk, or breathe
3. Severe stridor

4. Cyanosis
5. Extreme panic
6. Sternal retractions
7. Patient clutches throat with both hands (universal distress signal for airway obstruction)

Management

Conscious/responsive patient
Abdominal thrusts using the Heimlich maneuver

Unconscious/unresponsive patient
1. Activate EMS
2. **Begin CPR <u>without pulse check</u>**
3. Before ventilating check mouth for foreign object and remove.
4. Abdominal thrusts

Management of the Pregnant or obese patient

1. Perform chest thrusts from behind the patient. This can be performed while standing or kneeling.
2. **Do not perform abdominal thrusts!**

Management of the Infant

Conscious infant
1. Alternate 5 back blows with 5 chest thrusts

Unconscious infant
1. Send someone to activate EMS and begin CPR with no pulse check.
2. If alone, perform 5 cycles of CPR with no pulse check, and then activate EMS.

Practice Question 12
Which of the following signs may indicate complete airway obstruction?

A. Unable to cough, talk, or breathe
B. Has forceful cough

C. Extreme panic
D. Both A and C

Answers
A. Incorrect. Inability to cough, talk, or breathe is not the only sign of complete airway obstruction in this list.
B. Incorrect. A patient able to cough forcefully does not have a complete airway obstruction
C. Incorrect. Extreme panic is not the only sign of complete airway obstruction in this list.
D. Correct. Extreme panic and the inability to cough, talk, or breathe are signs of complete airway obstruction.

Practice Question 13
While performing the Heimlich maneuver on a choking patient, the patient loses consciousness and is lowered to the floor. What should the respiratory therapist do NEXT?

A. Begin CPR
B. Check for a pulse
C. Blind finger sweep of the airway
D. Abdominal thrusts

Answers
A. Correct. You may begin CPR without checking for a pulse in the unconscious choking victim.
B. Incorrect. Checking for a pulse is not necessary prior to giving CPR in this case.
C. Incorrect. A blind finger sweep may push the object deeper into the patient's airway, making the situation worse. However, you may visually inspect the mouth and remove any foreign objects prior to ventilating the patient.
D. Incorrect. Abdominal thrusts are not indicated at this point.

Tracheal Intubation

Indications

AARC guidelines list over 40 specific indications for endotracheal intubation. Rather than memorizing them all, focus instead on the following **four general guidelines** for intubation.

1. **Impending or actual respiratory failure**
2. **Airway compromise**
   - A. Burns and edema to the face and neck
   - B. Epiglottitis
   - C. Severe stridor
3. **Airway protection**
   - A. Drug overdose
   - B. Dysphagia in the stroke or dementia patient
   - C. Meconium stained amniotic fluid
4. **Emergency medication** (given through the ETT during CPR)
   - A. Epinephrine
   - B. Versed
   - C. Atropine
   - D. Narcan

Exam Tip: Patient's without IV access can be given <u>Epinephrine, Narcan, Versed, and Atropine</u> through the endotracheal tube. Give twice the normal intravenous dose and then flush the ETT with 10 mL of saline.

Complications

Complications of intubation are too numerous to memorize. The following complications are the most likely to be encountered on the exam.

1. Right mainstem intubation
2. Laryngospasm
3. VAP (Ventilator Associated Pneumonia)

4. Vocal cord damage
5. Tracheal stenosis
6. Tracheal malacia

Contraindications

1. Do not resuscitate (DNR) order
2. Do not intubate (DNI) order

Airway Anatomy

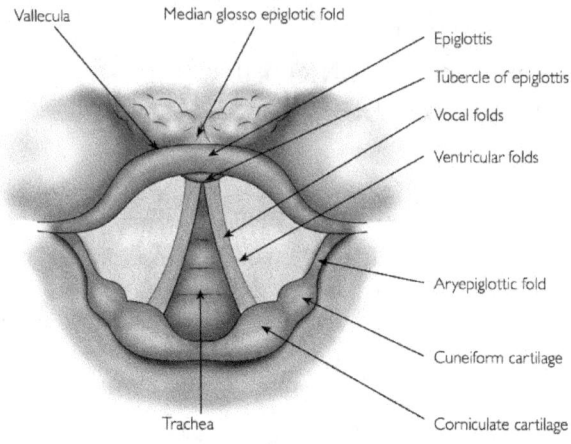

Epiglottis
The epiglottis covers and protects the glottic opening. The epiglottis is lifted out of view during laryngoscopy with the Miller blade.

Vallecula
The vallecula is a depression located just behind the root of the tongue. The Macintosh blade is inserted into the vallecula during laryngoscopy.

Vocal folds
Vocal folds are the proper term for vocal chords.

Endotracheal Intubation Equipment
Laryngoscope
Handle
Bulb
Batteries

Blades
Either the Macintosh or Miller blade may be used for endotracheal intubation. Selection of either blade is dependent upon the clinician's personal preference.

Macintosh
Macintosh is a curved blade. Remember: The "c" in the word Macintosh is curved like the blade.

Miller
Helpful way to remember: Remember: The "l" in the word Miller is straight like the blade.

Blade Size

Adult	3-4
Child	2
Full Term Infant	1
Pre Term Infant	0

Endotracheal Tube Size

Adult Male	8.0-9.5 mm
Adult Female	7.0-8.0 mm
Full Term Newborn 38-42 weeks	3.0 to 4.0 mm
Pre-Term Newborn <37 weeks	2.5 to 3.0 mm

Stylet
A Stylet provides rigidity to the ETT allowing it to be shaped or angled as needed.

Bag valve-mask
A bag valve-mask (BVM) is necessary to provide manual ventilation before and after endotracheal intubation. The BVM

depends on many working parts and proper user technique to be effective.

ETCO2 detector

Disposable end tidal CO2 detectors or continuous waveform end tidal CO2 analysis provide confirmation of tube placement by detecting the presence of carbon dioxide.

Syringe

Connect to the pilot balloon to inflate the endotracheal tube cuff.

Lubrication

Water based lubricant can be placed on the tip of the ETT to reduce friction during insertion.

Endotracheal Intubation Procedure

A. Gather and assemble equipment
B. Position patient in sniffing position with head only slight hyperextended
C. Pre oxygenate and ventilate
D. Hold laryngoscope in left hand
E. Insert the laryngoscope blade into the right side of the mouth, sweeping the tongue from right to left.

    1. <u>Macintosh blade</u> – The Macintosh blade is curved and inserted into vallecula to indirectly raise epiglottis.
    2. <u>Miller blade</u> – The Miller blade is straight and inserted under the epiglottis to lift it directly.

F. <u>Insert tube</u>

	Tube Insertion Depth
Endotracheal intubation	21 to 25 cm at the lip
Nasotracheal intubation	26 to 29 cm at the nares

G. <u>Inflate cuff</u>

1. Minimal leak technique. Cuff is inflated until no air leak is heard and then deflated until a slight leak is heard at peak inspiration.
2. Minimal occluding volume. Cuff is inflated until no air leak is heard at peak inspiration.
3. Cuff pressure can be measured using a cufflator, or combining a syringe, three-way stopcock, and pressure manometer.
4. Recommended cuff pressure is 20 – 25 mm Hg, or 25 – 35 cm H20.

H. Assess tube position
   1. Observe chest rise – Normal is symmetrical.
   2. Auscultation – Normal bilateral, equal breath sounds.
   3. Capnometry – Yellow color indicates presence of CO2.
   4. Chest X-ray – The tip of the ETT should reside 2 to 5 cm above the carina or at the aortic knob as viewed on the chest X-ray.

I. Stabilize/secure the ETT

Exam Tip: Weak batteries will cause the bulb to appear yellowish or dim. Check and change if necessary prior to procedure.

Exam tip: A high cuff pressure will cause damage to the tracheal wall. Inflating the cuff too little may cause aspiration of secretions. Inflate the cuff to the recommended cuff pressure.

Exam Tip: Troubleshoot bulb failure in this order:
1. Tighten bulb
2. Check if blade is attached
3. Change blade
4. Check batteries

Exam Tip: Flexion or extension of the head will change the position of the endotracheal tube.

Nasotracheal Intubation
Indications

1. Maxillofacial or dental surgery
2. Limited ability to open mouth
3. Severe swelling of the tongue

Complications
1. Epistaxis (nose bleed).
2. Similar to endotracheal intubation
3. Sinusitis

Contraindications
1. DNR/DNI
2. Basilar skull fracture
3. Patients with coagulopathies

Equipment
1. Magill forceps – Used to lift tube into trachea during nasal intubation.
2. Use smaller size tube than oral route
3. Water soluble lubricant

Nasotracheal intubation procedure
1. Anesthetize the nose.
2. Lubricate the tube with water-soluble lubricant.
3. Use Magill forceps to guide the tube into the airway.
4. Insert tube 26-29 cm at patient's nares.

Exam Tip: When manually ventilating a patient with a bag-valve device, suspect a leak if no resistance or chest rise is observed while squeezing the bag.

Exam Tip: Position the stylet at least 1 cm away from the tip of the ETT to prevent injury to the patient's airway. Bend the opposite end of the stylet at the top of the ETT so that it cannot advance through the ETT resulting in trauma.

Practice Question 14

The endotracheal tube cuff pressure of an adult male ICU patient reads 38 mm Hg. The patient weighs 75 Kg, is 68 inches tall and has a size 8.0 ETT. What should the therapist do NEXT?

A. Re-intubate the patient with a larger ETT
B. Deflate the cuff until it measures 20 mm Hg
C. Deflate the cuff using the minimal occluding volume technique and reassess.
D. Deflate the cuff until it measures 25 cm H20

Answers

A. Incorrect. The size 8.0 ETT is appropriate for an adult male patient.
a. Incorrect. This is within the recommended cuff pressure range, however, setting the cuff at a predetermined pressure without assessing its effectiveness is not advisable.
b. Correct. Use the minimal amount of pressure necessary to occlude the area around the ETT at peak inspiration.
c. Incorrect. Ideal cuff pressure serves as a guideline only. Airway protection is of greater importance.

Difficult Airway

A difficult airway is one in which an experienced provider cannot effectively provide mask ventilation and/or tracheal intubation. As a result, multiple laryngoscopy attempts may lead to airway trauma and swelling. A critical airway event may result in which the provider can neither mask ventilate the patient nor intubate the patient.

The NBRC will test your knowledge regarding difficult airway recognition and management.

Signs of Potential Difficult Airway
1. Patients with short or asymmetric necks
2. Obese patients
3. Overbite
4. Pregnant patients

Difficult Airway Management

Sellick maneuver
The Sellick maneuver is the application of firm external pressure to the cricoid cartilage. The proposed benefit of this maneuver is to bring an anterior airway into view. This maneuver may also prevent air from entering the esophagus and regurgitation of gastric contents during bag-valve-mask ventilation.

LMA
Difficult to bag-mask ventilate or intubate patients may benefit from placement of an LMA. Some LMA's allow passage of an ETT through them without removing the LMA.

King Airway
The King airway is indicated as an <u>out of hospital emergency airway</u> in patients who are difficult to bag-mask ventilate or

intubate. King airways are discussed in more detail in the Supraglottic airway chapter.

Esophageal Tracheal Combitube (ETC)

The ETC is indicated as an <u>out of hospital emergency airway</u> in patients who are difficult to bag-mask ventilate or intubate. The ETC is placed blindly into the trachea or esophagus. The ETC is discussed in more detail in the Supraglottic airway chapter.

Cricothyroidotomy

Cricothyroidotomy is performed emergently in "can't intubate, can't ventilate" patients. A cricothyroidotomy may be performed surgically or with the use of a needle. A surgical cricothyroidotomy creates an incision in the cricothyroid membrane through which a tracheostomy tube or endotracheal tube can be passed. Needle cricothyroidotomy uses a 14-gauge needle advanced through the cricothyroid. Regardless of the method used, a cricothyroidotomy is performed as a last resort method to establish a patent airway.

Percutaneous Trans Tracheal Jet Ventilation

Percutaneous trans tracheal jet ventilation is used to provide ventilation to a patient post cricothyroidotomy.

Exam Tip: Recommend neuromuscular blocking agents such as succinylcholine to induce short-term paralysis during intubation attempts.

Airway Exchange Catheters

Airway exchange catheters can be used to exchange an endotracheal tube, or to secure the airway should the patient fail extubation and require re-intubation.

Bougie
The bougie (also known as gum-elastic bougie or introducer) is advanced into the endotracheal tube. The ETT is then removed while the bougie catheter is left in place. The new ETT is then railroaded over the bougie catheter. The bougie catheter has no central lumen for oxygen insufflation.

Cook AEC
The Cook airway exchange catheter is used in a similar manner to the bougie; however, it has a central lumen and 15 mm adaptor for oxygen insufflation.

Extubation

Complications
1. Laryngospasm
2. Laryngeal edema
3. Airway obstruction
4. Vocal cord paralysis

Procedure
1. Perform a qualitative leak test. Deflate cuff, observe at least 15% decrease in exhaled tidal volume.
2. Gather equipment: Syringe, yankeur, oxygen, bag-valve mask, equipment for re-intubation.
3. Minimize risk of hypoxemia by pre-oxygenating patient.
4. Suction the artificial and oropharyngeal airway.
5. Fully deflate cuff
6. Instruct patient to take a full deep breath.
7. Remove tube at peak inhalation or when patient coughs.

Exam Tip: If the patient is unstable following extubation; re-intubate the patient.

      A. Severe stridor – re-intubate
      B. Mild stridor, stable vital signs – try racemic epinephrine, cool aerosol.

Decannulation

Decannulation is the removal of the tracheostomy tube from the patient's airway. Timing of decannulation varies depending upon why the patient received a tracheostomy in the first place. For example, a patient requiring tracheostomy to bypass a mass obstructing the airway will be treated differently than a patient recovering from prolonged mechanical ventilation due to respiratory failure.

Care of the stoma

Following decannulation, the stoma can be cleaned using a cotton tip applicator with a 50/50 hydrogen peroxide and water solution. Dress the stoma with sterile gauze. Antibiotic creams can be applied if signs of infection appear.

General guidelines

1. Cuff deflation trial
2. Change to fenestrated tracheostomy tube
3. Speaking valve trial
4. Capping trial 24 to 72 hours

Practice Question 15

While assessing an adult patient on mechanical ventilation, the respiratory therapist notes gurgling sounds coming from the patient's mouth. The cuff pressure measures 23cm H20 and the ETT is secured at 23 cm at the lip. What should the therapist do NEXT?

    A. Advance the ETT
    B. Suction the airway
    C. Add air to the cuff
    D. Re-intubate the patient

Answer

    A. Incorrect. There is no evidence the ETT needs to be advanced. Normal depth of insertion is between 21 and 26 cm at the lip for the adult population.

B. Incorrect. This is a good answer, but not the best. Because the cuff pressure of 23cm H20 is lower than recommended cuff pressure guidelines, an underinflated cuff should be suspected.
C. Correct. . Because the cuff pressure of 23cm H20 is lower than recommended cuff pressure guidelines, an underinflated cuff should be suspected.
D. Incorrect. Re-intubation is not indicated.

Practice Question 16

The exhaled tidal volume on an adult patient receiving volume control ventilation has decreased from 550 ml's to 450 ml's. Breath sounds are equal and the ETT is secured at 22 cm at the lip. What should the therapist do NEXT?

A. Advance the ETT
B. Add air to the cuff
C. Suction the patient
D. Order a chest X-ray

Answer
A. Incorrect. 22cm is a normal insertion depth for an adult patient.
B. Correct. Adding air to the cuff will prevent air from escaping around the ETT.
C. Incorrect. Secretions in the airway will not cause loss of volume in a patient on volume control ventilation.
D. Incorrect. A chest X-ray could help identify the ETT position, however, this will take too long and is not the best answer

Airway Clearance Techniques

Maintaining a patent airway is important for both the artificial and natural airway.
Mobilization and removal of airway secretions can decrease airway resistance and improve oxygenation and ventilation.

Bronchial Hygiene Devices & Maneuvers

Postural drainage
Postural drainage uses the force of gravity to mobilize retained secretions.

Manual percussion/chest physiotherapy
Manual percussion involves clapping on the patient's chest with cupped hands. The clapping transmits vibrations through the chest wall, which mobilizes the secretions. Manual percussion should be followed by deep breathing and coughing by the patient to clear the mobilized secretions from the lungs.

Vibratory PEP
Vibratory PEP is an excellent airway clearance device that can be used by both inpatient and outpatient populations to facilitate airway clearance.

Recommend for patients with bronchiectasis as part of a pulmonary hygiene program. Vibratory PEP has an advantage over manual percussion because it does not require a trained caregiver to administer.

HFCWO
High frequency chest wall oscillation loosens and mobilizes airway secretions. HFCWO is contraindicated in patients with head and neck injury.

Recommend HFCWO for:
1. Patients who have no caregiver to provide manual percussion.
2. Patients too fragile for manual percussion,

3. Patients with a history of multiple exacerbations or hospital admissions.
4. Patients with bronchiectasis, cystic fibrosis, and chronic bronchitis.

Insufflation/exsufflation device

These devices inflate the lungs using positive pressure and then simulate a cough using negative pressure. Insufflation/exsufflation devices are also known as cough assist devices or mechanical insufflation-exsufflator (MIE) devices. Recommend for patients with neuromuscular diseases such as cerebral palsy.

Huff cough maneuver

The huff cough maneuver is useful to clear mucus from the smaller airways. With the huff cough maneuver, the patient takes a deep breath and exhales forcefully but slowly while keeping the vocal chords open. The procedure is repeated up to four or five times. Care must be taken to not exhaust the patient performing the huff cough maneuvers.

Quad cough maneuver

The patient takes a deep breath in and coughs. At the moment the patient coughs, the therapist gently pushes upward and inward on the patient's abdomen. This creates enough force to help the patient expectorate the secretions. The quad cough maneuver is recommended for patients with central nervous system disorders such as spinal cord injury.

Mucolytics

Patients with persistently thick, retained secretions, such as with cystic fibrosis, may benefit from aerosolized mucolytics such as acetylcysteine (Mucomyst), or Pulmozyme.

Exam Tip: Recommend vibratory PEP to patients following chest surgery, rather than manual percussion. Manual percussion should not be performed on patients following surgery of the chest due to tenderness and pain surrounding the incision sites.

Suctioning

Indications
1. Stimulate cough
2. Clear secretions
3. Sputum sample collection

Complications/hazards
1. Hypoxemia
2. Bradycardia and PVC's may occur due to hypoxemia or vagus nerve stimulation
3. Trauma
4. Bronchospasm
5. Infection
6. Atelectasis may occur when suctioning with a catheter greater than half the internal diameter of the artificial airway.

Suctioning Routes

Oropharyngeal Suctioning
Be sure to use a different catheter when suctioning the lungs after suctioning the mouth.

Nasotracheal Suctioning
Place the patient in the sniffing position. Watery secretions are a sign the catheter entered the esophagus or stomach.

Artificial Airway Suctioning
The natural airway in the healthy patient is cleared and maintained by waves of cilia and a strong cough. Cilia are found in the epithelial cells extending from the bronchioles to the trachea. When the patient's airway is bypassed with an artificial airway, it loses its ability to clear secretions.

Suctioning Equipment

Closed suction catheter systems reduce the risk of oxygen desaturations, arrhythmias, and infection as compared to open systems. Closed systems allow mechanically ventilated patients to continue receiving ventilation and oxygen during the procedure.

Open suction catheters require disconnection from the mechanical ventilator. This causes loss of PEEP and exposes the patient's airway to contamination and infection. This potentially exposes the patient to outside pathogens. In addition, the subsequent loss of PEEP can produce negative outcomes.

Catheter sizing
The ideal suction catheter should be no more than half the internal diameter of the airway. Suction catheters are measured in French units. French sized suction catheters are available in even numbered sizes: 4, 6, 8, 10, 12, 14, and 16.

Choose the correct size French suction catheter by multiplying the ETT by 2 and then choosing the next size down.

For a size 8.0 ETT, multiply 8 x 2, which = 16. Then select the next size lower, which is 14 Fr.

ETT Size	French Catheter Size
8.0 mm	14 Fr
7.0 mm	12 Fr
6.0 mm	10 Fr
5.0 mm	8 Fr

Vacuum Pressure
The vacuum pressure should be set according to the following guidelines.

Adult	-100 to -120 mm Hg
Child	-80 to -100 mm Hg
Infant	-60 to -80 mm Hg

Exam Tip: If the therapist is having trouble suctioning an artificial airway despite using the correct size catheter, the vacuum pressure may be set too low.

Coude tipped catheter

Coude tipped suction catheters have an angled tip to direct the catheter into the left mainstem bronchus.

Turning the patient's head can also facilitate suctioning of the left or right mainstem bronchus when using a non-coude tipped catheter. For example, turning the patient's head to the right side will cause the suction catheter to enter the left mainstem bronchus.

Saline instillation
Saline instillation may be useful for removing tenacious secretions, however, it may also increase the amount of secretions. Cough, bronchospasm, and airway irritation are also side effects of saline instillation. Therefore, it should not be performed routinely for all patients.

Heat and Humidification
Heat and humidification are important to prevent drying of secretions. Heat is important to prevent dysfunction of the cilia. Thickening of secretions, known as inspissation, can also occur if adequate humidification is not provided.

Exam Tip: Tracheostomy patients with thick, difficult to suction secretions may benefit from a heated aerosol rather than a cool aerosol system.

Bronchoscopy

Rigid bronchoscopy
Recommend to remove foreign bodies from the airway.

Flexible bronchoscopy
Recommend for removal of retained secretions and as an aid in the diagnosis of cancer or infection. Pictures, washings, and samples of the lung can be obtained using diagnostic bronchoscopy

Mucus shaver

The mucus shaver is a catheter designed to remove secretions stuck to the inside of the endotracheal tube.

Airway Emergencies Common to Children

Foreign body aspiration

Foreign body airway obstruction is common among **young children**. Recommend rigid bronchoscopy to clear aspirated objects.

Signs
1. Sudden onset
2. Violent cough
3. Cyanosis
4. Retractions

Exam Tip: Aspirated objects are often radiolucent. As a result, they <u>will not be visible on a chest X-ray.</u> Inspiratory and expiratory chest X-rays may reveal air trapping on the side of the aspirated object.

Epiglottitis

Epiglottitis is an airway emergency caused by supraglottic swelling (above the vocal cords). Epiglottitis is commonly caused by Haemophilus influenza B infection. On chest X-ray the epiglottis appears thick and flat with a characteristic thumb sign.

Exam Tip: Do not stimulate patient or visually inspect airway.

Croup

Croup causes subglottic swelling and is common in children 6 months to 6 years old. Croup is caused primarily by a viral infection and is characterized by a barking cough and a steeple sign on lateral neck X-ray.

Exam Tip: Managing Stridor

Epiglottis, croup, and foreign body aspiration can all cause stridor. Stridor is a high-pitched, monophonic sound made as air passes through a narrowed glottic opening.

1. Patient is unstable with severe or marked Stridor – Intubate
2. Patient is stable with mild or moderate stridor – Recommend racemic epinephrine, cool aerosol, corticosteroids, obtain lateral neck X-ray.

Exam Tips Summary

1. Do not perform head-tilt/chin-lift if spinal trauma suspected. For example, motor vehicle accidents, falls. Instead, use the modified jaw thrust maneuver.

2. Do not recommend oropharyngeal airways for conscious or semi-conscious patients.

3. A BVM is a required piece of equipment when transporting intubated patients and when performing a cardioversion.

4. If the BVM is equipped with a reservoir bag, increase oxygen flow to the bag if it does not refill in between delivering each breath.

5. A leak anywhere in the BVM system may cause poor chest rise and/or a lack of resistance when squeezing the bag.

6. Epinephrine, Narcan, Versed, and Atropine can be given through the endotracheal tube in patients lacking IV access. Give twice the normal intravenous dose and then flush the ETT with 10 mL of saline.

7. Severe or marked Stridor, unstable = Intubate

8. Mild or moderate stridor, stable = racemic epinephrine, cool aerosol, obtain lateral neck X-ray

9. Troubleshoot bulb failure in this order: Tighten bulb, check blade is attached, change blade, and check batteries.

10. Weak batteries will cause the laryngoscope bulb to appear yellowish or dim. Check and change if necessary prior to intubation.

11. The stylet should be at least 1 cm away from the tip of the ETT to prevent injury to the patient's airway. The opposite end of the stylet should be bent so that the stylet cannot inadvertently advance too far through the ETT.

12. Some exam questions require you to troubleshoot equipment. However, this can sometimes be a trap. If an option exists to simply get another piece of equipment, this is usually the better answer. An exception would be to increase the flow to a reservoir bag that is not inflating after each breath.

13. If a bag valve-mask device malfunctions, replace it. Do not attempt to fix it.

14. A high cuff pressure will cause damage to the tracheal wall. Inflating the cuff too little may cause aspiration of secretions. Inflate the cuff to the recommended cuff pressure of 20 – 25 mm Hg, or 25 – 35 cm H20.

15. Flexion or extension of the head will change the position of the endotracheal tube.

16. Recommend neuromuscular blocking agents such as succinylcholine to induce short-term paralysis in patients with a difficult airway.

17. The King airway and esophageal tracheal combitubes (ETC) are not intended for long-term ventilation and should be replaced with an endotracheal tube as soon as possible.

18. Recommend a double-lumen endobronchial tube for independent lung ventilation.

19. When deciding if a patient needs to be reintubated consider the overall stability of the patient. If the patient has stable vital signs you may try to treat them with medications such as racemic epinephrine. If the patient has unstable vital signs they should be immediately reintubated.

20. Manual percussion should not be performed on patients following surgery of the chest due to tenderness and pain surrounding the incision sites. Recommend vibratory PEP to patients following chest surgery, rather than manual percussion.

21. Minimizing hypoxemia when suctioning is important to the NBRC. Steps you can take to minimize hypoxemia include pre-oxygenating the patient prior to the procedure. Use closed system suction catheters on mechanically ventilated patients. Limit suctioning procedure to 15 seconds or until complications occur; whichever occurs first. Stop suctioning when any complications occur

22. If the therapist his having trouble suctioning an artificial airway despite using the correct size catheter, the vacuum pressure may be set too low.

23. Tracheostomy patients with thick, difficult to suction secretions may benefit from a heated aerosol rather than a cool aerosol system.

24. Aspirated objects are often radiolucent. As a result, they will not be visible on a chest X-ray. Inspiratory and expiratory chest X-rays may reveal air trapping on the side of the aspirated object.

25. Do not stimulate or visually inspect the airway of an epiglottis patient.

Practice Exam Questions

1. Which of the following devices are used to directly lift the epiglottis during endotracheal intubation?

   A. Magill forceps
   B. Miller blade
   C. LMA
   D. Macintosh blade

2. Immediately following endotracheal intubation a disposable capnometer changes color from purple to yellow. This color change most likely indicates the ETT is?

   A. In the esophagus
   B. In the right mainstem bronchus
   C. In the airway
   D. Kinked

3. An oropharyngeal airway is placed in a lethargic patient to maintain a patent airway. The patient begins to cough and gag. The respiratory therapist should?

   A. Reassure the patient
   B. Continue to monitor the patient
   C. Remove the oropharyngeal airway
   D. Intubate the patient

4. After changing a mechanically ventilated patient's tracheostomy tube, the patient's breathing becomes labored. Substernal retractions are visible and subcutaneous emphysema is palpated around the airway. What should the therapist doe NEXT?

   A. Order a chest X-ray
   B. Call the attending physician
   C. Order an arterial blood gas
   D. Remove the airway and ventilate the patient with a bag and mask.

5. To reduce damage to the tracheal mucosa the maximum recommended cuff pressure is?

   A. 25 mm Hg or 35 cm H20
   B. 40 mm Hg or 45 cm H20
   C. 15 mm Hg or 25 cm H20
   D. 10 mm Hg or 20 cm H20

6. Contraindications to LMA insertion include?

   A. Elective surgery
   B. Risk of aspiration
   C. Patient who is spontaneously breathing
   D. Difficult to ventilate with bag and mask

7. Which of the following steps during manual bag mask ventilation will help ensure the highest delivered oxygen level?

   A. Use a flow rate of 10 to 15 LPM
   B. Deliver breath over 1 second
   C. Use bag with an oxygen reservoir
   D. All of the above

8. The correct order for assessing ETT position immediately post intubation is?

   A. Capnography, auscultation, observe rise and fall of chest, chest X-ray
   B. Observe rise and fall of chest, auscultation, capnography, chest X-ray
   C. Chest X-ray, auscultation, capnography, observe rise and fall of chest
   D. Observe rise and fall of chest, chest X-ray, capnography, auscultation

9. Which of the following items are not necessary when preparing equipment for nasotracheal intubation?

   A. Bag-valve mask
   B. Stylet

C. Magill forceps
D. Disposable capnometer

10. Which of the following maintains patency of the stoma following decanulation?

    A. Nasopharyngeal airway
    B. Oropharyngeal airway
    C. Tracheostomy button
    D. Trans tracheal catheter

11. The respiratory therapist is called to assess a tracheostomy patient with labored respirations. Upon arrival the therapist notes a SPo2 of 83% on .35 Fio2 cool aerosol collar. The therapist is unable to pass a suction catheter through the tracheostomy tube. What should the therapist do FIRST?

    A. Increase the FiO2
    B. Change the tracheostomy tube
    C. Manually ventilate the patient's tracheostomy tube
    D. Use a smaller suction catheter

12. A respiratory therapist is having difficulty suctioning an adult patient in the ICU. The therapist is using a size 14 French catheter to suction a size 8.0 ETT. The vacuum pressure is set to 80 mm Hg. What should the therapist do NEXT?

    A. Increase vacuum pressure
    B. Use larger catheter
    C. Instill mucolytic
    D. Use a smaller catheter

13. A conscious patient in the ICU has a large amount of secretions they are unable to clear due to an ineffective cough. They require frequent naso-tracheal suctioning. Which of the following airways should the respiratory therapist recommend?

A. Oropharyngeal airway
B. Nasopharyngeal airway
C. Postural drainage
D. Chest physiotherapy

14. A patient has just been extubated to a cool aerosol mask with a FiO2 of .28. The patient develops severe stridor, and sub-sternal retractions. The Spo2 is 80% and the pulse is 120 bpm. What should the therapist recommend NEXT?

A. Re-intubation
B. Increase the FiO2
C. Mask CPAP
D. Nebulized racemic epinephrine

15. Immediately following intubation, breath sounds are decreased on the left side and increased on the right. This most likely indicates?

A. Left mainstem intubation
B. Right mainstem intubation
C. Pneumothorax
D. Pneumonia

16. Esophageal intubation will reveal a capnometer reading of?

A. 0%
B. 3%
C. 5%
D. 40%

17. The respiratory therapist uses the minimal occluding volume technique to adjust a patient's endotracheal tube cuff pressure. The therapist then measures the 6.0 ETT cuff pressure at 40 mm Hg. What should the therapist recommend NEXT?

A. Replace the ETT with a larger one

B. Remove air from the cuff until the pressure is 20 mm Hg
C. Use the minimal leak technique
D. Nothing, 40 mm Hg is normal

18. The most appropriate airway for a patient with severe facial trauma is?

A. Endotracheal tube
B. Nasotracheal tube
C. Tracheostomy tube
D. LMA

19. Which of the following artificial airways should the respiratory therapist recommend for the prevention of VAP in the adult patient receiving mechanical ventilation?

A. CASS tube
B. Combitube
C. Dual lumen tube
D. Guedel airway

20. After administering 8 abdominal thrusts to a choking patient, the patient is still conscious and still has an obstructed airway. What should the therapist do NEXT?

A. Stop treating and observe the patient
B. 5 back blows
C. Chest compressions
D. Continue abdominal thrusts

21. While suctioning a patient in the ICU, the respiratory therapists notes the following rhythm:

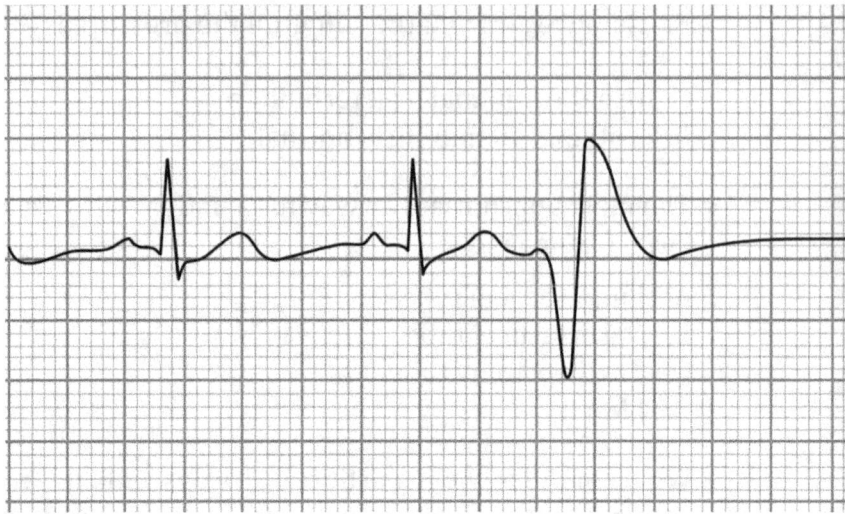

What should the therapist do NEXT?

A. Stop suctioning
B. Increase the FiO2
C. Increase the PEEP level
D. Give Epinephrine

22. A king airway has which of the following features?

A. Two lumens
B. Single lumen and two cuffs
C. Single lumen and one cuff
D. Two lumens and one pilot balloon

23. The esophageal tracheal combitube has which of the following features?

A. Two lumens, two cuffs, and two pilot balloons
B. One lumen, one cuff, and one pilot balloon
C. Two lumens, one cuff, and one pilot balloon
D. Two lumens, one pilot balloon, and two cuffs

24. The maximum recommended vacuum pressure used for suctioning the adult patient is?

A. 80 mm Hg
B. 120 mm Hg

C. 140 mm Hg
D. 60 mm Hg

25. A tracheostomy patient in the ICU has not required mechanical ventilation for the past 48 hours. The patient is awake and alert. What should the respiratory therapist recommend to begin weaning the patient from the tracheostomy tube?

A. Change to a foam filled cuffed tracheostomy tube.
B. Deflate the cuff for 3 days
C. Change to a fenestrated tracheostomy tube
D. Change to a Jackson tracheostomy tube

Practice Questions With Rationales

1. Which of the following devices are used to directly lift the epiglottis during endotracheal intubation?

   A. Magill forceps
   B. Miller blade
   C. LMA
   D. Macintosh blade

   Answers
   A. Incorrect. Magill forceps are used to lift the nasotracheal tube during nasotracheal intubation.
   B. Correct. The Miller blade is inserted directly beneath the epiglottis and lifts it out of the way of the glottic opening.
   C. Incorrect. The LMA sits above the epiglottis.
   D. Incorrect. The Macintosh blade is inserted into the vallecula to indirectly lift the epiglottis.

2. Immediately following endotracheal intubation a disposable capnometer changes color from purple to yellow. This color change most likely indicates the ETT is?

   A. In the esophagus
   B. In the right mainstem bronchus
   C. In the airway
   D. Kinked

   Answers
   A. Incorrect. Carbon dioxide should not be present in the esophagus.
   B. Incorrect. The capnometer cannot differentiate which mainstem the endotracheal tube is in.
   C. Correct. Presence of carbon dioxide in the lungs will change the capnometer from purple to yellow.

D. Incorrect. A kinked ETT will not allow carbon dioxide to flow through the capnometer. Thus, the color will not change from purple to yellow.

3. An oropharyngeal airway is placed in a lethargic patient to maintain a patent airway. The patient begins to cough and gag. What should the respiratory therapist do NEXT?

   A. Reassure the patient
   B. Continue to monitor the patient
   C. Remove the oropharyngeal airway
   D. Intubate the patient

   Answers
   A. Incorrect. Reassuring the patient will not control the patient's gag reflex and puts the patient at risk of vomiting and aspirating.
   B. Incorrect. Continuing to monitor the patient will not control the patient's gag reflex and puts the patient at risk of vomiting and aspirating.
   C. Correct. Oropharyngeal airways are contraindicated in patients with an intact gag reflex.
   D. Incorrect. A lethargic patient is not an indication for intubation. The therapist should remove the oropharyngeal airway first, and then consider a nasopharyngeal airway.

4. After changing a mechanically ventilated patient's tracheostomy tube, the patient's breathing becomes labored. Substernal retractions are visible and subcutaneous emphysema is palpated around the airway. What should the respiratory therapist do NEXT?

   A. Order a chest X-ray
   B. Call the attending physician
   C. Order an arterial blood gas
   D. Remove the airway and ventilate the patient with a bag and mask.

   Answers

A. Incorrect. This patient is unstable and needs an immediate intervention. A chest X-ray will take too long to obtain.
B. Incorrect. This patient is unstable and needs an immediate intervention. Calling the attending physician will take too long.
C. Incorrect. Arterial blood gas provides no value in this airway emergency.
D. Correct. The patient's airway is most likely displaced. The patient is unstable and needs an immediate intervention. Removing the airway and ventilating with a bag and mask is the best choice.

5. To reduce damage to the tracheal mucosa the maximum recommended cuff pressure is?

   A. 25 mm Hg or 35 cm H20
   B. 40 mm Hg or 45 cm H20
   C. 15 mm Hg or 25 cm H20
   D. 10 mm Hg or 20 cm H20

   Answers
   A. Correct.
   B. Incorrect.
   C. Incorrect.
   D. Incorrect.

6. Contraindications to LMA insertion include?

   A. Elective surgery.
   B. Risk of aspiration.
   C. Patient who is spontaneously breathing
   D. Difficult to ventilate with bag and mask

   Answers
   A. Incorrect. Elective surgery is often performed using an LMA.
   B. Correct. The LMA does not protect the airway from aspiration.

C. Incorrect. Spontaneously breathing patients may be managed with an LMA as long as they are properly anesthetized.
D. Incorrect. LMA's are indicated for patients who are difficult to ventilate with a bag and mask. Keep in mind the patient must be properly anesthetized or unconscious to use the LMA.

7. Which of the following steps during manual bag mask ventilation will help ensure the highest delivered oxygen level?

A. Use a flow rate of 10 to 15 LPM
B. Deliver breath over 1 second
C. Use bag with an oxygen reservoir
D. All of the above

Answers
A. Incorrect.
B. Incorrect.
C. Incorrect.
D. Correct. All of these maneuvers ensure delivery of the highest possible oxygen level during bag mask ventilation.

8. The correct order for assessing ETT position immediately post intubation is?

A. Capnography, auscultation, observe rise and fall of chest, chest X-ray
B. Observe rise and fall of chest, auscultation, capnography, chest X-ray
C. Chest X-ray, auscultation, capnography, observe rise and fall of chest
D. Observe rise and fall of chest, chest X-ray, capnography, auscultation

Answers
A. Incorrect.
B. Correct.

C. Incorrect.
D. Incorrect.

9. Which of the following items are not necessary when setting up for nasotracheal intubation?

   A. Bag-valve mask
   B. Stylet
   C. Magill forceps
   D. Disposable capnometer

   Answers
   A. Incorrect.
   B. Correct. A stylet is not used for nasotracheal intubation.
   C. Incorrect.
   D. Incorrect.

10. Which of the following maintains patency of the stoma following decannulation?

    A. Nasopharyngeal airway
    B. Oropharyngeal airway
    C. Tracheostomy button
    D. Trans tracheal catheter

    Answers
    A. Incorrect. Nasopharyngeal airways are only inserted into the patients nares.
    B. Incorrect. Oropharyngeal airways are only inserted into the patients mouth.
    C. Correct. A tracheostomy button is a short, hollow tube used to maintain the patency of a stoma following decannulation.
    D. Incorrect. A trans tracheal catheter will not maintain the patency of a stoma following decannulation.

11. The respiratory therapist is called to assess a tracheostomy patient with labored respirations. Upon arrival the therapist notes a SPo2 of 83% on .35 Fio2 cool aerosol collar. The therapist is unable to pass a suction

catheter through the tracheostomy tube. What should the therapist do FIRST?

A. Increase the FiO2
B. Change the tracheostomy tube
C. Manually ventilate the patient's tracheostomy tube
D. Use a smaller suction catheter

Answers
A. Incorrect. Increasing the FiO2 will not benefit a patient with an airway obstruction.
B. Correct. The patient's tracheostomy tube is obstructed and should be removed immediately.
C. Incorrect. The tracheostomy tube is obstructed and cannot be ventilated.
D. Incorrect. A smaller suction will not relieve the obstruction.

12. A respiratory therapist is having difficulty suctioning an adult patient in the ICU. The therapist is using a size 14 French catheter to suction a size 8.0 ETT. The vacuum pressure is set to 80 mm Hg. What should the therapist do NEXT?

A. Increase vacuum pressure
B. Use larger catheter
C. Instill mucolytic
D. Use a smaller catheter

Answers
A. Correct. The maximum recommended vacuum pressure for suctioning an adult patient is 120 mm Hg.
B. Incorrect. The size 14 French catheter is appropriate for an 8.0 ETT.
C. Incorrect. Using a mucolytic to may be recommended only after all other measures are attempted.
D. Incorrect. A smaller suction catheter may make it more difficult to suction retained secretions in this adult patient.

13. A conscious patient in the ICU requires frequent naso-tracheal suctioning. Which of the following airways should the respiratory therapist recommend?

    A. Oropharyngeal airway
    B. Nasopharyngeal airway
    C. Postural drainage
    D. Chest physiotherapy

    Answers
    A. Incorrect. An oropharygeal airway does not facilitate nasotracheal suctioning.
    B. Correct. A nasopharyngeal airway will help reduce trauma to the nares of a patient requiring frequent nasotracheal suctioning.
    C. Incorrect. Postural drainage may help mobilize secretions. However, it will not improve the patient's ability to expectorate and clear them.
    D. Incorrect. Chest physiotherapy may help mobilize secretions. However, it will not improve the patient's ability to expectorate and clear them.

14. A patient has just been extubated to a cool aerosol mask with a FiO2 of .28. The patient develops severe stridor, and sub-sternal retractions. The Spo2 is 80% and the pulse is 120 bpm. What should the therapist recommend NEXT?

    A. Re-intubation
    B. Increase the FiO2
    C. Mask CPAP
    D. Nebulized racemic epinephrine

    Answers
    A. Correct. The patient is unstable and requires immediate re-intubation.
    B. Incorrect. Increasing the FiO2 will not relieve the patient's stridor and substernal retractions. These are signs of airway compromise. The patient's airway must be secured without delay.

C. Incorrect. Mask CPAP is not recommended for patients with airway compromise.

D. Incorrect. This patient is unstable and needs an immediate intervention. Administering racemic epinephrine will delay care of this unstable patient.

15. Immediately following intubation, breath sounds are decreased on the left side and increased on the right. This most likely indicates?

A. Left mainstem intubation
B. Right mainstem intubation
C. Pneumothorax
D. Pneumonia

Answers
A. Incorrect. Left mainstem intubation would reveal increased breath sounds on the left as compared to the right.

B. Correct. Right mainstem intubation is a common complication of endotracheal intubation.

C. Incorrect. Pneumothorax is possible, however, in the context of the procedure that was just performed it is not the most likely or best answer.

D. Incorrect. There is no indication the patient has pneumonia. In addition, pneumonia would reveal bronchial breath sounds over the affected lung.

16. Esophageal intubation will reveal a capnometer reading of?

A. 0%
B. 3%
C. 5%
D. 40%

Answers
A. Correct. Carbon dioxide should not be present in the esophagus.

B. Incorrect.

C. Incorrect.
D. Incorrect.

17. The respiratory therapist uses the minimal occluding volume technique to adjust a patient's endotracheal tube cuff pressure. The therapist then measures the 6.0 ETT cuff pressure at 40 mm Hg. What should the therapist recommend NEXT?

   A. Replace the ETT with a larger one
   B. Remove air from the cuff until the pressure is 20 mm Hg
   C. Use the minimal leak technique
   D. Nothing, 40 mm Hg is normal

   Answers
   A. Correct. A cuff requiring a higher than recommended pressure to achieve the minimal occluding volume indicates the tube may be too small.
   B. Incorrect. 20 mm Hg is recommended, however, 40 mm Hg is required to achieve the minimal occluding volume.
   C. Incorrect. The minimal leak technique will allow microaspiration of secretions.
   D. Incorrect. 40 mm Hg is too high of a pressure to apply against the tracheal wall.

18. The Most appropriate airway for a patient with severe facial trauma is?

   A. Endotracheal tube
   B. Nasotracheal tube
   C. Tracheostomy tube
   D. LMA

   Answers
   A. Incorrect. The oral route of intubation should be avoided in patient's with severe facial trauma.
   B. Incorrect. Nasal intubation should be avoided in patient's with severe facial trauma.

C. Correct. A tracheostomy tube can be inserted and secured in patient's with severe facial trauma.
D. Incorrect. The LMA is contraindicated for use in patient's with severe facial trauma.

19. Which of the following advanced artificial airways should the respiratory therapist recommend for the prevention of VAP in the adult patient receiving mechanical ventilation?

A. CASS tube
B. Combitube
C. Dual lumen tube
D. Guedel airway

Answers
A. Correct. CASS tubes provide continuous aspiration of subglottic secretions.
B. Incorrect. The combitube does not provide a mechanism to aspirate subglottic secretions.
C. Incorrect. The dual lumen tube does not provide a mechanism to aspirate subglottic secretions.
D. Incorrect. The Guedel airway is a pharyngeal airway only.

20. After administering 8 abdominal thrusts to a choking patient, the patient is still conscious and still has an obstructed airway. What should the therapist do NEXT?

A. Stop treating and observe the patient
B. 5 back blows
C. Chest compressions
D. Continue abdominal thrusts

Answers
A. Incorrect. Continue abdominal thrusts until the airway is cleared or the patient becomes unconscious.
B. Incorrect. Back blows are not performed on the adult patient.

C. Incorrect. Chest compressions are not indicated on the conscious patient.

D. Correct. Continue abdominal thrusts until the airway is cleared or the patient becomes unconscious.

21. While suctioning a patient in the ICU, the respiratory therapists notes the following rhythm:

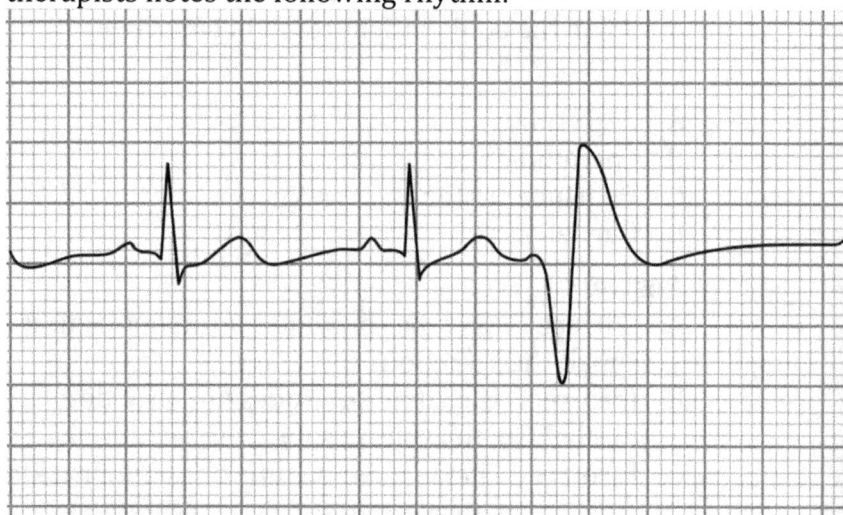

What should the therapist do NEXT?

A. Stop suctioning
B. Increase the FiO2
C. Increase the PEEP level
D. Give Epinephrine

Answers

A. Correct. Premature ventricular contractions may result from stimulation of the vagus nerve, or hypoxemia. Stop the procedure immediately.

B. Incorrect. The patient may need more oxygen, however, the procedure should be stopped first.

C. Incorrect. Increasing the PEEP may have a detrimental effect on the patient's hemodynamics. Stopping the procedure is the best answer.

D. Incorrect. Premature ventricular contractions are not treated with epinephrine.

22. A king airway has which of the following features?

    A. Two lumens
    B. Single lumen and two cuffs
    C. Single lumen and one cuff
    D. Two lumens and one pilot balloon

    Answers
    A. Incorrect.
    B. Correct. The King airway has a single lumen and two cuffs.
    C. Incorrect.
    D. Incorrect

23. The esophageal tracheal combitube has which of the following features?

    A. Two lumens, two cuffs, and two pilot balloons
    B. One lumen, one cuff, and one pilot balloon
    C. Two lumens, one cuff, and one pilot balloon
    D. Two lumens, one pilot balloon, and two cuffs

    Answers
    A. Correct. The ETC has two lumens, cuffs, and pilot balloons.
    B. Incorrect
    C. Incorrect
    D. Incorrect

24. The maximum recommended vacuum pressure used for suctioning the adult patient is?

    A. 80 mm Hg
    B. 120 mm Hg
    C. 140 mm Hg
    D. 60 mm Hg

    Answers
    A. Incorrect
    B. Correct. 120 mm Hg is the maximum recommended vacuum pressure for suctioning the adult patient.
    C. Incorrect

D. Incorrect

25. A tracheostomy patient in the ICU has not required mechanical ventilation for the past 48 hours. The patient is awake and alert. What should the respiratory therapist recommend to begin weaning the patient from the tracheostomy tube?

    A. Change to a foam filled cuffed tracheostomy tube.
    B. Deflate the cuff for 3 days
    C. Change to a fenestrated tracheostomy tube
    D. Change to a Jackson tracheostomy tube

    Answers
    A. Incorrect. Part of the weaning process may include the use of a cap or speaking valve. A foam filled cuff cannot be used with a cap or speaking valve.
    B. Incorrect. The cuff should have already been deflated when mechanical ventilation was discontinued.
    C. Correct. A fenestrated tracheostomy tube reduces resistance to airflow in non-ventilated patients and allows air to pass through the vocal chords, nose and mouth.
    D. Incorrect. Jackson tracheostomy tubes are not recommended for patients weaning from a tracheostomy tube. Jackson tracheostomy tubes are only rarely used for patients requiring long-term tracheostomy tubes.

More By The Author

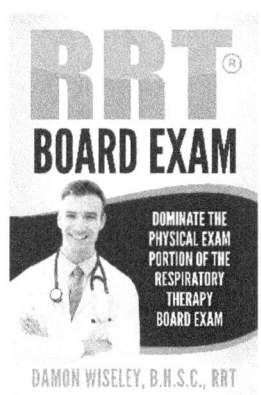

Available at: http://www.amazon.com/dp/B01BM0AK3S

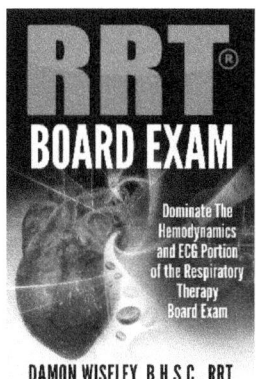

Available at: http://www.amazon.com/dp/B01FQ0WGXW

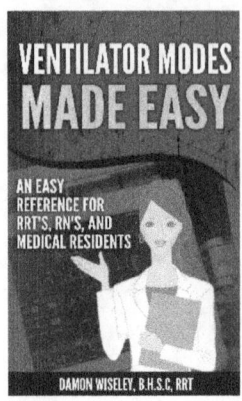

Available at: http://www.amazon.com/dp/B00P085K5C

I really hope you liked this book. Let's be honest; I hope you loved it! But, just in case you didn't, I'd love to hear from you. Tell me what could make this book better. What do you feel I may have missed?

Here is my personal email: respprograms@gmail.com. Let me know what you think. Tell me the good, the bad, and the horrible. This will only help me make better products for YOU and, other respiratory therapists/students out there.

I'm hard at work on the next book in this series. To get a free preview of the next book before it is released, sign up to my subscriber newsletter at www.respiratorytherapyprograms.com.

References

Agrò F, Frass M, Benumof J, Krafft P, Urtubia R, Gaitini L, Giuliano I. *Minerva Anestesiol.* The esophageal tracheal combitube as a non-invasive alternative to endotracheal intubation. *A review.* 2001 Dec; 67(12):863-74.

Hess, D. R., Kacmarek, R. M. Essentials of Mechanical Ventilation, 2014. 3rd edition. McGraw Hill.

Heur, A. J., Scanlan, C. L. 2014. *Wilkins' Clinical Assessment in Respiratory Care.* 7th edition. Mosby.

Kacmarek, R. M., Stoller, J. K., Heuer, A. J., (2013) *Egan's Fundamentals of Respiratory Care.* 10th edition. Elsevier.

www.ingramcontent.com/pod-product-compliance
Lightning Source LLC
Chambersburg PA
CBHW060405190526
45169CB00002B/763